SHYANN MCK

Thrive Beyond 40

Your Guide to Staying Fit, Finding Joy, and Redefining Wellness After 40

Contents

Introduction

Although turning 40 is frequently referred to as the beginning of a new chapter, for many women, it can be the start of an unwanted tale. You're enjoying your life, and suddenly it feels like your energy, health, and social circle have been dealt a one-way ticket to decline. I understand how it feels. I have also been there. And it affects all of us, not just you.

The majority of women begin to notice significant changes in their 40s. One day you're feeling great, and the next you're dealing with a sore body, constant exhaustion, and the depressing realization that you've changed. Social life?

It should come as no surprise that it appears to be vanishing as well. It feels that those pals who used to be around constantly are now just acquaintances. This transition occurs for a variety of reasons, but one thing is certain: these changes are significant and real.

The good news is that every shift we experience is a door, and we can choose how to respond to it. I can assure you that we are halfway to feeling better once we begin to examine the reasons behind these changes. Ignoring it or attempting to "tough it out" simply makes us feel more powerless and alienated. We must stop pondering the reason and begin taking action to recover our vitality, social lives, and our well-being.

In this book, we shall directly address these trends. More importantly, I'll teach you how to handle everything with courage and composure. I'll walk you through your physical and mental processes. This is not just about surviving; it's about thriving. We might reconsider what well-being after 40 means if we are aware of what is going on both inside and outside of us.

So, collectively, let's set off on this expedition. Because you won't just get by after your forties; you'll thrive.

Chapter 1: Understanding Midlife Changes

Section 1: Physical Changes in Midlife

When we hit our 40s, our bodies start going through changes that can feel as surprising as they are frustrating. One day, it's smooth sailing; the next, it's like everything we thought we knew about our bodies is flipped upside down. These shifts are real, and they're often rooted in three big changes: hormones, metabolism, and sleep.

Hormonal Shifts

Hormones are the body's natural messengers, and in our 40s, they start sending us some pretty mixed messages. For many women, this is the time when estrogen and progesterone levels begin to fluctuate as part of perimenopause, leading to a whole host of unexpected symptoms. These hormonal shifts can lead to mood swings, hot flashes, and even changes in energy levels that feel completely out of character.

As women approach their 40s, they experience significant hormonal changes, which play a central role in the transformations occurring within their bodies. Hormones like estrogen, progesterone, and testosterone begin to fluctuate, and these shifts can impact everything from physical health to emotional stability.

Understanding the reasons behind these hormonal changes and the effects they produce can be empowering, helping us take control of our well-being during this period.

The Role of Estrogen

Estrogen is often called the primary female hormone, and it is a powerhouse when it comes to our health. It supports everything from reproductive health and strong bones to a happy heart and clear thinking. But as women enter perimenopause and estrogen levels start to decline, we can notice some pretty significant changes. You might experience hot flashes, night sweats, or changes in your skin—like less collagen, which can lead to a bit of sagging and dryness.

This hormone also has a big impact on how we feel mentally. Because estrogen is linked to serotonin, the "feel-good" neurotransmitter, a drop in estrogen can lead to mood swings and even increased anxiety. You might find yourself feeling a bit less sharp mentally, which can be frustrating!

Plus, let's talk about heart health. Estrogen plays a crucial role in keeping our cholesterol levels in check and our blood vessels nice and flexible. So when estrogen levels dip, it can raise our risk for issues like high blood pressure, weight gain, and high cholesterol. That's why it's especially important to keep an eye on heart health during this time.

Progesterone Fluctuations

In addition to estrogen, progesterone is another important hormone that starts to decline as we enter midlife. Often recognized for its calming effects, progesterone plays a key role in helping us get a good night's sleep. So, when progesterone levels drop, many women find themselves struggling with insomnia and other sleep issues.

With this drop in progesterone, you might notice feeling more emotionally sensitive, a bit more irritable, or even experiencing spells of sadness. It's as if the soothing influence of progesterone has faded away, leaving us feeling a bit more on edge.

Progesterone also works closely with estrogen to help regulate our menstrual cycles. When progesterone levels fall, our cycles can become a bit unpredictable. Some women might experience shorter or longer cycles, and periods can become heavier or more painful. These shifts are often early signs of perimenopause and can be a gentle reminder to prioritize some extra self-care during this transitional time.

Testosterone in Women

Even though testosterone is often thought of as a male hormone, it's really important for women's health too, especially for things like muscle tone, energy, and sex drive. As women get older, their testosterone levels can drop, which may lead to lower muscle tone, less energy, and in some cases, even a decrease in bone density.

Many women have a sensation of sluggishness as a result of this testosterone reduction, with less energy for physical activity. Because testosterone affects sexual desire and response, it also has an impact on libido.

This shift may have an effect on relationships or self-esteem for certain people. Women who are aware of these changes can start to adjust by exercising, eating a healthy diet, and being honest with their relationships.

Navigating Hormonal Shifts

The physical and emotional challenges that come with hormonal changes can feel quite overwhelming at times. However, these shifts also highlight how important it is to focus on self-care. Eating a balanced diet filled with whole foods, especially those containing phytoestrogens like soy, can help reduce some of those uncomfortable symptoms.

Staying active is just as crucial. Regular exercise, particularly weight-bearing and resistance workouts, supports your bone and muscle health. Don't overlook mindfulness practices, either! Activities such as meditation can greatly enhance your emotional well-being.

For some women, hormone replacement therapy (HRT) might be a helpful option. It can provide relief from symptoms like hot flashes, sleep problems, and mood swings. That said, it's a personal decision, so it's a good idea to discuss it with your healthcare provider to understand the potential benefits and risks.

You might also consider natural supplements like black cohosh, evening primrose oil, or maca root. Many women find these helpful for managing symptoms such as hot flashes or mood changes. Just remember to consult your healthcare provider before starting any new supplement routine, as natural approaches often require patience and consistency.

Hormonal changes are a natural part of a woman's life journey, bringing both challenges and opportunities. By understanding the causes and effects of these changes, women can adapt more easily and take on new practices that help them feel strong, empowered, and resilient through midlife and beyond.

Mood and Emotional Health

Hormonal changes during midlife are closely tied to how we feel emotionally. As estrogen levels drop, which is directly linked to serotonin (the neurotransmitter that helps regulate our mood), many women start to notice mood swings, increased anxiety, and even feelings of sadness.

This decrease in estrogen can also affect how we think, impacting memory and clarity. You might find yourself forgetting things more often or struggling to concentrate, which can be disconcerting. It's important to remember that these changes are completely normal and part of the hormonal transition.

Progesterone plays a key role in helping us feel balanced and calm. When its levels fluctuate, you might experience heightened irritability or emotional sensitivity. By recognizing that these feelings are simply a natural part of the hormonal changes we go through, you can lessen self-criticism and create space for lifestyle adjustments that promote emotional well-being.

Energy Levels and Fatigue

Along with mood changes, many women in midlife find that their energy levels drop and they feel more tired overall. Hormones like testosterone, which help keep our energy up and our motivation strong, gradually decrease during this time. This can leave some women feeling less lively and less able to handle daily tasks.

Additionally, sleep quality may deteriorate when progesterone and estrogen levels drop. Common concerns like insomnia, trouble falling asleep, or waking up without feeling rejuvenated can further sap vitality and negatively affect general health. The exhaustion that results can be discouraging, particularly for women who are accustomed to being highly active or productive.

Practices like consistent, restful sleep, mindful diet, and regular exercise can help strengthen stamina and reduce some of the frequent symptoms of exhaustion, even if these energy swings are a normal part of the hormonal transition.

Weight and Body Composition

Hormonal changes during midlife can really affect weight and body shape, creating some new challenges for many women. As estrogen levels start to drop, you might notice that your body tends to redistribute weight, often around the tummy area. This shift can come along with a slower metabolism, which means it might be easier to gain weight and trickier to lose it compared to before.

Testosterone, which helps keep muscle mass intact, also decreases, and that can lead to less muscle tone and a higher percentage of body fat. It's understandable to feel a bit down about these changes, especially if the methods that used to work for managing your weight aren't as effective anymore.

But don't worry! Adding strength training to your routine, enjoying a balanced diet that includes plenty of protein, and staying active can help tackle these changes. Remember, these shifts are a normal part of life and not just a result of lifestyle choices, so being gentle with yourself as you navigate this phase is important.

While these hormonal shifts in mood, energy, and body composition can be significant, they also present a great chance for self-care and reassessing your wellness practices. By keeping yourself informed about these natural changes, you can face midlife with confidence, adjusting your routines and habits to better support your evolving needs.

Metabolism and Weight Gain

Another big factor in changes during midlife is our metabolism. Metabolism is how our body turns food into energy, and as it starts to slow down, we might find it easier to gain weight, even if our diet and activity level stay the same. This can feel frustrating, but knowing why this happens can help us manage it better.

Why Metabolism Slows

The slowing of metabolism, which can begin as early as the 30s but becomes more visible around age 40, is one of the most obvious consequences of hormonal changes. This drop in metabolic rate is directly caused by a decrease in hormones such as testosterone and estrogen.

Testosterone promotes muscular growth, while estrogen is crucial in controlling the distribution of body fat. At rest, muscle burns more calories than fat, therefore when testosterone levels drop, muscular tissue gradually disappears, which lowers the body's capacity to burn calories.

The body's energy needs decrease when muscle mass gradually decreases, so maintaining weight or energy levels may no longer be achieved with the same diet and exercise regimen.

Impact on Weight and Energy Levels

As metabolism slows down, gaining weight can become easier, especially around the belly. The drop in estrogen and slower metabolism both play a role in how our bodies store fat, and many women find they gain extra fat in their stomach area. This change is common but can be frustrating.

Having extra weight can affect how we look and also lower our energy levels since carrying more weight makes physical activities harder and can lead to tiredness, especially when hormonal changes disrupt our sleep.

When energy levels drop, it's common to be less active, which can create a cycle that leads to more weight gain and fatigue. While this shift is completely natural, women need to see it as a normal part of midlife, not as a personal failure.

Dietary Adjustments for Metabolism

While hormonal shifts and metabolic changes are a natural part of life, making some dietary adjustments can help support a more efficient metabolism and keep your energy levels up. Eating a balanced diet that includes lean proteins, healthy fats, and complex carbohydrates can make a big difference.

Lean proteins—like chicken, fish, legumes, and tofu—are vital for maintaining muscle mass, which is crucial for a healthy metabolism. By adding more protein to meals and snacks, women can help counteract muscle loss and boost their metabolic rate.

Healthy fats from sources like avocados, nuts, seeds, and olive oil provide sustained energy and can help manage cravings that may arise due to hormonal fluctuations. Complex carbohydrates, such as whole grains, sweet potatoes, and leafy greens, offer a steady release of energy, preventing those pesky blood sugar spikes and crashes that can sap your energy.

In addition to focusing on these nutrient-rich foods, eating smaller, more frequent meals can help stabilize blood sugar levels and maintain consistent energy throughout the day. Staying hydrated is also super important—just mild dehydration can affect how well your metabolism functions.

Many women also find that cutting back on processed foods and added sugars helps with weight management. These foods can cause insulin spikes, which can make it easier to gain weight. By understanding how hormonal changes influence metabolism, women can adjust their eating habits to better align with their body's needs.

Facing the challenges of a slower metabolism and shifting energy levels in midlife calls for a kind and adaptable approach. By prioritizing nutrient-dense foods, staying hydrated, and being mindful of portion sizes, women can support their metabolism and energy levels, turning these hormonal changes into a chance for renewed health and self-care.

Sleep and Recovery Challenges

Once we reach our 40s, a good night's sleep can start to feel like a rare treat. Whether it's hormonal shifts, rising stress levels, or changes in sleep patterns, midlife often presents its unique sleep challenges that can impact our recovery, mood, and overall well-being.

Challenges with Falling and Staying Asleep

As estrogen and progesterone levels decline, many women find it increasingly difficult to fall asleep and stay asleep. Estrogen plays a crucial role in regulating body temperature, which is essential for falling asleep comfortably. When estrogen levels drop, it can lead to night sweats and hot flashes that disrupt sleep, making it hard to find that cozy position to drift off or to get back to sleep after waking up.

At the same time, progesterone—a hormone that naturally helps us relax—also decreases. This can leave us feeling less able to unwind and settle into a restful sleep. As a result, sleep patterns can become more fragmented, with many women waking up multiple times during the night and struggling to reach that deep, restorative sleep that we all need to feel our best.

Quality of Sleep Affects Recovery

Sleep quality plays a huge role in how we feel physically, mentally, and emotionally. During those deep sleep phases, our bodies do important work—repairing tissues, processing memories, and restoring energy. This stage is especially vital for women in midlife, as it supports overall health and resilience.

When sleep is fragmented or insufficient, it can throw off this recovery process. Many women find themselves feeling tired, mentally foggy, and less equipped to handle stress the next day. Plus, not getting enough deep sleep can weaken the immune system and contribute to inflammation, making it easier to get sick and harder to bounce back from physical activities.

These sleep challenges are often made worse by hormonal changes that can affect metabolism, leading to an increased risk of weight gain, less muscle tone, and lower energy levels. By recognizing the connection between hormonal shifts, sleep quality, and overall recovery, we can take proactive steps to enhance our wellness and feel our best.

Tips to Improve Restorative Sleep

While those hormonal changes can really throw a wrench in our sleep, the good news is there are some effective strategies to help you snag more restful and restorative slumber. Creating a relaxing bedtime routine can work wonders for both your body and mind.

Try simple things like dimming the lights, cutting down on screen time an hour before bed, and enjoying calming activities like reading or doing some gentle stretches. These little rituals signal to your body that it's time to wind down. And don't forget about your bedroom environment! Keeping it cool and comfy can help manage those pesky hot flashes or night sweats, making it easier to enjoy uninterrupted sleep.

Your food choices can also play a big part in how well you sleep. If you can, try to reduce your caffeine in the afternoon, cut back on alcohol, and add some magnesium-rich goodies like leafy greens, nuts, and seeds. They can really help you relax and improve the depth of your sleep.

And let's not overlook physical activity! Gentle, consistent exercise can do wonders for lowering stress levels and keeping your body's internal clock on track.

If sleep still feels like it's playing hard to get, don't worry! You can also explore mindfulness and relaxation techniques. Deep breathing, progressive muscle relaxation, or even guided meditation can help ease your mind into that calm, restful state.

By embracing these habits in response to hormonal shifts, you can approach sleep with a lot more confidence. Here's to getting the restful, restorative sleep you need to thrive through midlife and beyond!

Section 2: Emotional and Psychological Shifts

The changes we experience in our bodies during midlife are just one part of the whole picture. This stage of life also brings emotional and mental shifts that can be just as strong, changing how we view ourselves, handle stress, and think about our mental health. Let's explore some of the main emotional changes many women go through, like redefining who they are, managing stress, and taking care of their mental well-being.

Self-Identity and Midlife

Midlife can change how we see ourselves. It's a time when many of us take a moment to think about who we are, where we've been, and where we want to go next. It's completely normal to feel a mix of pride, nostalgia, and even some uncertainty during this period.

Questioning Roles and Purpose

One of the biggest changes that comes with midlife is the chance to rethink who we are and what we want to do. Many women who have spent years taking care of others or focusing on their careers start to wonder about their own identity outside of those roles.

As hormones shift and feelings change, it's normal to ask ourselves where we fit in and what we want in this new phase of life. With kids becoming more independent and careers reaching a steady point, it's common to feel a bit lost or unsure. This can be a good time to explore what truly makes us happy.

Taking time to reflect is a great opportunity to reconnect with our interests and values. It helps us create a life that feels right for us and meets our personal goals. It's all about discovering what brings us joy and makes us feel good

Balancing Past and Future

Midlife can feel like standing at a crossroads, where we look back at what we've been through and think about what's ahead. The changes in our hormones might make us feel nostalgic or even a bit regretful, but they can also spark a wish to plan for a fresh and exciting chapter in life.

This time is all about finding a balance between accepting our past—both the ups and downs—and keeping a hopeful view of the future. While the experiences we've had offer us valuable lessons, it's also a chance to think about new opportunities that are waiting for us.

Finding this balance can feel empowering, helping women create a life that respects their past while looking forward with hope and confidence. It's a wonderful moment to think about where we've been and where we want to go next.

Redefining Self-Worth

As hormonal changes affect both our physical and emotional stability, many women start to rethink how they see their self-worth. For a long time, society has often defined a woman's value by her youth, productivity, or how she fits into others' lives. But midlife is a time when these outside measures often start to matter less.

During this phase, self-worth shifts from seeking validation from others to finding value within ourselves, focusing on qualities like resilience, wisdom, empathy, and self-acceptance. This change means letting go of the need for approval based on looks or achievements and recognizing the strengths and insights that come from life experience.

For many women, this time of redefining self-worth brings a deeper sense of confidence and appreciation for their unique journey. By focusing on inner strengths and respecting themselves, they can develop a richer perspective on life. Midlife becomes not just a continuation of the past but a celebration of who they are and the valuable contributions they bring to the world.

Stress and Burnout

By the time we hit our 40s, many of us have been juggling work, family, relationships, and personal goals for quite a while. This constant balancing act can lead to chronic stress and even burnout, which can affect our mental health if we don't take care of it.

Identifying Burnout Symptoms

Midlife burnout often feels much more intense than regular stress. It can leave you physically worn out, emotionally drained, and feeling detached from everything, which can be tough. Life's responsibilities combined with hormonal changes can make these feelings even stronger. Paying attention to early signs of burnout—like feeling tired all the time, being irritable, or feeling disconnected—can help you practice self-compassion and find your energy again.

Just taking a few minutes for yourself each day can make a big difference, allowing you to reconnect and recharge. And don't forget, it's perfectly okay to say "no" sometimes. Doing so can help you save your energy and focus on what really matters to you.

Managing Chronic Stress

Chronic stress can impact all areas of our lives, from how well we sleep to how our immune system works. During midlife, it's common for stress levels to rise due to added responsibilities or life changes, so finding ways to manage stress is really important for staying healthy and getting your energy back.

Practicing mindfulness techniques like meditation, deep breathing, or just taking a moment to relax can help reduce the physical effects of stress and keep cortisol levels in a healthy range.

Getting regular exercise is another great way to let go of stress and boost your mood with those feel-good endorphins. Plus, setting small, achievable goals each day can give you a sense of accomplishment and keep you motivated without feeling overwhelmed.

Building a Support System

Having a good support system is important as you adjust to this new chapter in life. When times get tough, talking to family or close friends who listen without judging can be both comforting and helpful. Sometimes, joining a support group with others going through similar experiences can provide a special place for understanding and sharing ideas.

If the stress of midlife feels too heavy to handle alone, talking to a counselor or therapist can give you valuable guidance. A counselor can provide you with specific tools to help you face these changes with confidence and strength.

Mental Clarity and Cognitive Health

As we go through midlife, it's important to keep our minds clear and healthy. Many women start to notice some changes in their memory, focus, or how sharp they feel, which can be surprising and sometimes frustrating. But the good news is that there are plenty of simple ways to keep our minds active!

Supporting Cognitive Health

Just like we take care of our bodies, we need to give our brains some regular exercise and good habits, too. Fun things like puzzles, reading, or trying out a new hobby can really help. Studies show that even small brain exercises can strengthen our brain connections and slow down memory loss as we age.

Eating well is another big part of supporting our brain health. Foods rich in omega-3 fatty acids—like fish, walnuts, and flaxseeds—are especially good for our brains. Making sure we include these foods in our meals can boost our memory and focus.

And don't forget how important sleep is. A good night's rest helps our brains recover, process what we've learned, and store memories. When we make sleep a priority, we can help our brain health and keep our minds clear and sharp.

Mindfulness for Mental Clarity

Midlife can often feel like a juggling act with many responsibilities, but practicing mindfulness can help clear the mind and bring back focus. Even taking just five minutes a day for mindful breathing can make a big difference in how we feel.

Mindfulness doesn't just help reduce stress; it can also boost our brainpower by easing mental clutter and making it easier to handle distractions. Simple deep breathing exercises are great when you're feeling overwhelmed; they can help reset your mind and keep you focused on the present moment.

Another great way to practice mindfulness is by keeping a gratitude journal. Writing down a few things you're thankful for each day helps shift your attention to the good things in life, which can lift your spirits and create balance during stressful times.

Managing Age-Related Brain Changes

You may observe certain changes in your memory or information processing speed throughout this stage of life. Even though this is rather common, taking some proactive measures will help you maintain mental acuity and activity.

Maintaining an active mental life is among the best things you can do. This can be as easy as reading books, taking up new interests, or working through brainteasers and puzzles. You can keep your brain active by doing things that test your ability to think. Your brain's connections are formed and strengthened by these kinds of workouts, which can improve your ability to think clearly in general.

Another crucial strategy to maintain mental fitness is to socialize. Participating in group activities or spending time with loved ones can have a significant impact. Engaging with others can improve your mood and give your brain good exercise, both of which are good for your general health.

Don't forget how important exercise is! Regular activity helps your brain work better by releasing good chemicals that can protect it from some of the downsides of getting older. Just taking a daily walk can boost both your physical and emotional health.

Staying active during your midlife years helps you feel energetic and think more clearly. So, whether you join a yoga class, participate in a book club, or simply chat with friends, these activities can all help keep your mind lively and healthy!

Section 3: Common Health Concerns to Watch For

Midlife brings many changes, and along with them, there are some important health issues we should pay attention to. It's a great time to think about our bone, heart, and skin health. Let's examine these areas and find ways to care for ourselves as we go through this stage of life.

Bone Health and Osteoporosis

As we age, our bones can become less dense, and the risk of osteoporosis—which weakens bones and increases the chance of fractures—can become more likely for women over 40. Taking care of our bone health now is essential for maintaining our strength and mobility as we age.

Understanding Bone Loss

Bone density usually reaches its highest point in early adulthood, but it starts to go down gradually as we age. The biggest drop often happens around menopause due to hormonal changes. When estrogen decreases during this time, bones can become weaker and more likely to break.

It's important to be aware of your personal risk factors, such as having a family history of osteoporosis, not being very active, or being underweight. Knowing these factors can help you take care of your bone health. Regular bone density tests, recommended by your doctor, can give you helpful information about how strong your bones are and catch any early signs of osteoporosis or other issues.

It's also good to understand how calcium and vitamin D affect bone health. Calcium is essential for building strong bones, and vitamin D helps your body absorb calcium. Both are important for keeping your bones healthy.

Strengthening Bones Through Diet and Supplements

Eating a diet rich in nutrients is one of the best ways to keep your bones healthy. Adding specific foods and supplements can help maintain and even improve bone density.

Foods high in calcium, like leafy greens, dairy products, and fortified alternatives, are great for building strong bones. Vitamin D is also important for bone health because it helps your body absorb calcium. You can get vitamin D from sunlight, certain foods like fatty fish, and supplements, especially if you live in places or seasons with less sunlight.

Magnesium is another important nutrient for bone health that people often overlook. You can find magnesium in foods like nuts, seeds, and whole grains. It works with calcium and vitamin D to support bone growth. By including these key nutrients in your diet, you can make your bones stronger and help prevent bone loss as you get older.

Exercise for Bone Strength

Staying active is important for keeping your bones strong and healthy, and weight-bearing exercises are especially good for this. Activities like resistance training, whether you use bands or light weights, help your bones grow stronger and improve bone density.

Regular exercises like walking, jogging, or climbing stairs also help because they make your bones work against gravity, which is great for building and keeping bone strength.

Balance exercises, such as yoga or tai chi, are also helpful. They improve your stability and can lower the risk of falls, which is a common worry as our bones get weaker with age.

By mixing these types of activities into your routine, you not only strengthen your bones but also boost your overall health, making it less likely for you to experience fractures and helping you enjoy a better quality of life as you get older.

Heart Health and Cardiovascular Concerns

Looking after your heart is really important in midlife since the risk of heart problems can go up as we age. Problems like high blood pressure, high cholesterol, and heart disease are more common in women over 40. Taking steps to care for your heart can improve your life.

Understanding Cardiovascular Risks

As we go through midlife changes, the chance of heart problems, like heart disease, can go up. When estrogen levels drop during menopause, it can affect cholesterol and blood pressure.

To keep your heart healthy, it's a good idea to check your blood pressure and cholesterol levels regularly. Routine check-ups can help catch any early signs of heart issues so you can deal with them quickly. It's also important to notice warning signs like chest pain, shortness of breath, or feeling more tired than usual, as these could mean there's a heart problem that you might miss otherwise.

Your family history is also important. If heart problems are common in your family, it could impact your heart health. Knowing your risk factors can help you make better choices to take care of your heart during midlife and beyond.

Dietary Choices for Heart Health

What you eat matters a lot to your heart. Picking the right

foods can help keep your cholesterol, blood pressure, and heart in good shape. Healthy fats, like the ones in olive oil, nuts, and avocados, can help bring down bad cholesterol. These good fats are much better than the unhealthy ones in many processed foods.

Eating lots of fiber from whole grains, fruits, and vegetables is also great for your heart. Fiber helps lower cholesterol and keeps your blood sugar steady. Trying to eat different kinds of these foods every day will help your heart and make you feel better overall.

Keeping an eye on your salt intake is important, too. Eating too much salt can raise your blood pressure, which isn't good for your heart. To keep it in check, try using less salt when cooking, avoid processed foods, and check food labels. This can help keep your heart healthy over time.

Heart-Healthy Lifestyle Habits

Keeping your heart healthy isn't just about eating well; staying active, managing stress, and getting good sleep are all important too. Regular exercise, like brisk walking, biking, or swimming, helps your heart stay strong and keeps your blood flowing. Try to get at least 150 minutes of moderate activity each week to help lower heart risks and build up your energy.

Managing stress is also key since ongoing stress can raise blood pressure and cause other issues. Taking time for relaxing activities, like deep breathing, short breaks, or even meditation, can make a big difference.

Getting enough good-quality sleep is just as important. Poor sleep can lead to problems like high blood pressure, weight gain, and higher blood sugar. Creating a calm bedtime routine and a comfortable sleep space can help your body rest and recharge, keeping your heart healthier in the long run.

Skin Health and Aging

We usually notice signs of aging on our skin first, like fine lines and less elasticity. Even though these changes are a normal part of getting older, there are simple ways we can take care of our skin to keep it healthy and looking good.

Effects of Aging on Skin

As we get older, our skin starts to lose some of its firmness and elasticity. Collagen and elastin, which are important proteins that help keep our skin strong and flexible, begin to decrease. This loss of support can make the skin look thinner, more fragile, and more likely to develop wrinkles and sagging.

Things in our environment, especially the sun, can speed up this aging process. UV rays can damage collagen, causing early lines, dark spots, and less elasticity in the skin. Some lifestyle choices, like smoking, can also hurt the skin by limiting blood flow and speeding up the loss of important proteins. Plus, not drinking enough water can make fine lines stand out more.

By being aware of these factors, using sun protection, and

drinking plenty of water, we can help lessen some of these effects and keep our skin looking healthier as we age.

Skincare Essentials for Mature Skin
    Creating a simple skincare routine is a great way to keep mature skin healthy and glowing. Start with a gentle cleanser that won't strip away your skin's natural oils, as harsh cleansers can lead to dryness and irritation.

To keep your skin hydrated, use a good moisturizer with ingredients like hyaluronic acid or ceramides. These help draw in moisture and keep it locked in, so your skin feels soft and smooth.

Adding a product with retinoids or peptides to your routine can also make a difference. These ingredients support collagen production, which helps keep skin firm and smooth. With a few regular steps, you can keep your skin looking healthy, hydrated, and refreshed.

Nutrition and Lifestyle for Healthy Skin
    What we eat and how we live have a big impact on our skin's health and look, just like any skincare product. Foods like berries, leafy greens, and nuts are rich in antioxidants, which help fight aging by protecting against free radicals.

Cutting down on sugar is a good idea because too much can damage collagen and cause more lines and wrinkles. Getting enough sleep is also really important for healthy skin. A good night's rest helps your skin heal, keeping it fresh and glowing.

With a balanced diet, healthy habits, and enough rest, you're giving your skin the support it needs to stay vibrant and healthy at any age.

Chapter 2: Reclaiming Energy and Vitality

Section 1: Nutrition for Sustained Energy

In midlife, keeping your energy levels up can be tough because of different physical and hormonal changes. But with the right food choices, you can support your energy throughout the day. Let's talk about how balancing proteins, fats, and carbohydrates, getting key vitamins and minerals, and staying hydrated can help you feel energized.

Balancing Macronutrients

It's important to balance your macronutrients—proteins, fats, and carbohydrates—to maintain steady energy. Each of these plays a key role: proteins help your muscles repair and grow, fats give you lasting energy, and carbohydrates are the main source of quick energy for your body.

To create balanced meals, try to include a protein source, healthy fats, and complex carbs in each one. For example, a breakfast with scrambled eggs (protein), avocado (healthy fat), and whole-grain toast (carbohydrate) is a great way to start your day.

For lunch, think about having a salad with grilled chicken, mixed greens, nuts, and a splash of olive oil. At dinner, you could enjoy salmon (protein), quinoa (carbohydrate), and steamed veggies (fiber and nutrients). Snacking on things like Greek yogurt with berries or hummus with veggies can also help keep your energy up and prevent crashes throughout the day.

Key Vitamins and Minerals for Midlife

As women go through midlife, some vitamins and minerals become important for staying healthy and keeping your energy up. Nutrients like vitamin D, calcium, magnesium, and B vitamins are essential for energy production, strong bones, and keeping hormones in balance.

When you're lacking certain nutrients, you might notice signs like feeling tired, having mood swings, or getting sick more easily. To make sure you're getting what you need, try to eat a diet that includes lots of fruits, vegetables, whole grains, lean proteins, and healthy fats. Foods such as leafy greens, fatty fish, nuts, and fortified dairy products are great sources of these important nutrients.

Some women might find it helpful to take supplements if their diet isn't enough. It's a good idea to talk to a doctor to see what you might need and the best way to get it.

Hydration and Detoxification

Drinking enough water is very important for keeping your energy up, staying focused, and feeling good overall. Even slight dehydration can make you feel tired, less focused, and not perform well, which can affect your daily life.

Drinking water throughout the day helps your body work well, and adding hydrating foods like cucumbers, oranges, and watermelon can give you an extra boost. Many people find it helpful to set reminders to drink water or keep a reusable water bottle close by to make it easier to stay hydrated.

Natural detox practices work well with staying hydrated, helping your body get rid of toxins, and improving digestion. Herbal teas are especially good for this. Teas like dandelion, ginger, peppermint, and green tea are full of antioxidants and other good things that support your liver and kidneys, which are important for filtering out waste.

For example, ginger tea can help with digestion and reduce bloating, while dandelion tea supports liver health and encourages kidney function. These herbal teas not only help detoxify your body but also add to your daily fluid intake.

In addition to drinking water and herbal teas, probiotics are another great help for detoxification. Probiotics improve digestion and help your body process and get rid of waste by supporting a healthy gut.

Foods like yogurt, kefir, sauerkraut, and kombucha are rich in probiotics, and taking a daily probiotic supplement can help keep your gut healthy. Probiotics also work well with fiber-rich foods like leafy greens, berries, and whole grains to promote regular bowel movements, which helps with detoxification.

Building a routine that includes drinking enough water, enjoying herbal teas, and adding probiotics can boost your energy and overall health. Together, these habits help cleanse your body and support important functions, making you feel more vibrant and focused. By prioritizing hydration and detoxification, women can create a strong foundation for lasting health and energy well into their 40s and beyond.

Section 2: Exercise and Physical Activity

When women reach midlife, staying active and exercising regularly becomes very important for good health and feeling energetic. Doing a mix of different exercises, like strength training, cardio, and flexibility work, can boost your energy and improve your life. This section looks at the benefits of each type of exercise and shares easy tips to help women enjoy life after 40.

Strength Training and Muscle Health

Muscle strength naturally declines with age, primarily due to hormonal shifts and a decrease in physical activity.

Losing muscle can affect your strength, metabolism, and energy. But adding strength training to your routine can help with this. Strength training helps build and keep muscle, and it also speeds up your metabolism, which can help you stay at a healthy weight and feel more energetic during the day.

You can begin with simple strength exercises using just your body, like squats, lunges, and push-ups. Resistance bands or light dumbbells are also great tools to help build muscle strength. Try to do strength training exercises at least two to three times a week, and make sure to work on all the major muscle groups for the best results.

Cardiovascular Fitness for Heart Health

Cardiovascular fitness is essential for women in midlife, as the risk of heart disease increases with age. Regular cardio exercise strengthens the heart, enhances circulation, and improves endurance, all of which support overall health and vitality.

Effective exercises for heart health include walking, jogging, cycling, swimming, and dancing, all of which promote cardio-vascular fitness, boost energy, and improve mood. For safe and effective cardio routines, aim for at least 150 minutes of moderate-intensity exercise per week, which can be broken down into manageable sessions, such as 30 minutes of brisk walking five times a week.

Incorporating Zone 2 exercise is particularly beneficial for heart health. Zone 2 refers to a level of low-to-moderate intensity exercise where you can still hold a conversation but are slightly out of breath. This range, often at 60-70% of the maximum heart rate, optimizes fat-burning, builds endurance, and strengthens the cardiovascular system without overwhelming the body.

Zone 2 exercises—like steady-state cycling, walking uphill, or light jogging—are less intense but highly effective for long-term heart health and energy management. Including at least two to three sessions of Zone 2 training per week can improve aerobic capacity and help your body utilize oxygen more efficiently.

Adding interval training—alternating between higher and lower intensities—can also elevate cardiovascular benefits and make workouts more engaging. Embracing a combination of Zone 2 exercise, moderate cardio, and occasional intervals provides a balanced, sustainable approach to cardiovascular fitness for women in midlife.

Flexibility and Mobility for Longevity

Flexibility is really important for keeping a good quality of life, especially as we get older. Being flexible helps us move better, lowers the risk of injuries, and improves our posture, all of which support our overall well-being.

Doing daily stretches can help improve flexibility and make everyday tasks easier and more enjoyable. Focus on stretching major muscle groups like your hamstrings, quadriceps, shoulders, and back. Activities like yoga and Pilates are also great for boosting flexibility while helping you relax and clear your mind.

Taking care of our joints is key for staying active in the long run. As we age, our joints can wear down, so it's important to support them with good nutrition. Eating foods high in omega-3 fatty acids, like salmon, flaxseeds, and walnuts, can help reduce inflammation and ease joint pain. These healthy fats keep our joints lubricated and help protect cartilage.

Besides omega-3s, getting enough vitamin D and calcium is crucial for bone health, which helps our joints too. Foods like leafy greens, fortified dairy products, and fortified plant-based milk are excellent sources of these nutrients.

Eating antioxidant-rich foods like berries, cherries, and dark leafy veggies can help fight oxidative stress that can cause joint inflammation and damage. Also, foods that boost collagen, such as bone broth, chicken skin, and collagen supplements, can help keep our joints strong and support cartilage repair.

Staying hydrated is important too, as water helps keep our joint tissues flexible. Drinking enough water throughout the day keeps our joints well-lubricated and working smoothly.

Getting involved in low-impact activities, staying active, and following a balanced diet that supports joint health are key ways to keep our mobility and independence. Simple changes, like adding fatty fish to your meals, snacking on nuts and seeds, or including a variety of colorful veggies in your diet, can make a big difference.

By focusing on flexibility, mobility, and joint health through exercise and good nutrition, women can enjoy more independence and a more active life as they thrive after 40.

Section 3: Boosting Mental and Emotional Energy

As we go through midlife, it's important to work on boosting our mental and emotional energy for better overall well-being. Managing stress, setting boundaries, and getting involved in creative activities can help improve how clear our minds feel and how we handle emotions. In this section, we'll look at some great ways to refresh your mental and emotional energy so you can shine during this exciting time in your life.

Mindfulness and Stress Reduction

Stress can weigh us down, making it tough to enjoy life every day. Mindfulness practices can be wonderful for managing stress and finding peace.

When you bring mindfulness into your daily routine, you learn to deal with stress better, which helps keep your mental energy up. Simple things like paying attention to your breath or doing a quick meditation can help you stay present.

A great way to practice mindfulness is through deep breathing. It helps your body relax and move away from feeling stressed. To try deep breathing, find a quiet place where you won't be disturbed.

Sit comfortably, close your eyes, and put one hand on your chest and the other on your belly. Take a slow, deep breath through your nose, letting your belly rise as you fill your lungs. You should feel your hand on your belly lift as you breathe in. Hold that breath for a moment, then slowly breathe out through your mouth, allowing your belly to fall. Try to make your exhale a little longer than your inhale to help you relax.

Keep this up for several breaths, and focus on how it feels. If your mind drifts off, gently bring your attention back to your breath. Even just five minutes of deep breathing can help calm your mind, lower your anxiety, and give you a boost of energy.

You can also use mindful breathing during your day-to-day activities. Take a few deep breaths before a meeting, while taking a break, or even when you're waiting in line.

Making these small changes can really help you feel more balanced, focused, and ready to tackle the day. By making mindfulness and deep breathing a regular part of your routine, you can handle stress more easily.

Creating Boundaries and Saying No

Setting boundaries is important for keeping your mind healthy and saving your emotional energy. When life gets busy with lots of responsibilities, it's easy to take on too much.

Learning to say no is not just a good skill; it's also necessary for taking care of your time and energy. Start by looking at what you are currently committed to and see where you feel stressed.

Here are some simple tips for setting boundaries: let others know your limits, focus on tasks that are important to you, and pay attention to when you need a break.

Figuring out how and when to say no is a skill that you can get better at over time. Try to calmly express your needs, whether it's saying no to an invitation or putting off a project. By setting boundaries, you create space for self-care and renewal, helping you focus on what matters to you.

Practical Examples for Saying No

Saying no can be challenging, but having prepared responses can help you set boundaries respectfully and effectively. Here are five examples to help you say no in different situations, allowing you to prioritize your well-being and commitments:

Declining an Extra Work Assignment

Example: "Thank you for considering me, but my current workload is already full. I won't be able to take on this additional assignment right now."

Turning Down a Social Invitation

Example: "I appreciate the invite, but I've had a busy week and need to recharge. Let's catch up soon—maybe next week?"

Refusing a Favor You Can't Commit To

Example: "I wish I could help, but my schedule is very tight at the moment. I hope you understand, and please let me know if I can help in another way in the future."

Declining to Attend an Unnecessary Meeting

Example: "I believe my current projects will need my full attention, so I won't be able to join this meeting. Could you share the key points afterward?"

Saying No to Taking on Someone Else's Responsibilities

Example: "I'm focusing on my priorities right now, so I won't be able to take on this task. It may be helpful to find someone else who has the time to assist."

Hobbies and Creative Outlets

Getting involved in hobbies and creative activities can boost your mental health, especially during midlife. Being creative brings feelings of happiness, satisfaction, and purpose, helping you recharge your emotional energy.

Finding old hobbies that you love can be a great way to improve your well-being. Whether you enjoy painting, gardening, writing, or playing music, setting aside time for these activities lets you explore your passions and relieve stress.

Making time for these hobbies might need some planning, but even spending just a few minutes a day can make a big difference. Try to schedule specific times each week to enjoy your hobbies or try out new activities that interest you.

Enjoy the act of creating without worrying about being perfect—this approach can lift your spirits and help you find balance and joy in your life. By making creativity and self-expression a priority, you'll create a fuller, happier life that helps you thrive after 40.

Hobbies for Midlife

- **Gardening**: Caring for plants helps you relax and gives you joy as you watch them grow.
- **Photography**: Photography lets you be creative and gives you a reason to discover new places.
- **Cooking and Baking**: Cooking is a fun way to express yourself and enjoy making and tasting tasty meals.
- **Yoga and Meditation**: Activities like yoga or exercise help improve both your body and mind.
- **Reading and Book Clubs**: Reading can be relaxing, and joining a book club adds a social element to it.
- **Painting or Drawing**: Crafting is a calming way to express yourself, no matter if you're a beginner or have been doing it for years.
- **Dancing**: Dance classes are enjoyable and also a great way to meet new people.
- **Traveling**: Traveling to different places or cultures brings excitement and new experiences.
- **Learning a New Language**: Learning something new keeps your mind active and helps you connect with others.
- **Knitting or Crafting**: DIY projects let you make things you can use or give as gifts, while also helping you relax.
- **Writing or Journaling**: Writing can help you think about your life, or you might even start a blog or write a memoir.
- **Playing an Instrument**: Playing an instrument can be a fun challenge that helps your brain stay active while also being relaxing and energizing.
- **Hiking or Walking**: Being active outdoors not only helps you stay fit but also lets you enjoy the beauty of nature.
- **Volunteering**: Volunteering gives you a sense of purpose

and helps you connect with your community by giving back.

- **Puzzles or Board Games**: Puzzles and board games are a great way to keep your mind engaged and are even more fun when you play with friends or family.

Chapter 3: Building Lasting Healthy Habits

Section 1: Developing a Sustainable Routine

Creating a steady routine is important for staying healthy and full of energy as you go through midlife. A good routine brings stability to your life, encourages positive habits, and helps you feel better overall. In this section, we'll talk about why having a helpful morning and nighttime routine is essential, along with the advantages of keeping track of your progress to stay on track with your wellness journey.

Morning Routines for a Positive Start

Having a simple morning routine can help you start your day on the right foot, making you feel more energized and focused. A morning routine isn't just about getting things done; it also helps clear your mind and build emotional strength.

A good morning routine could include things like stretching or doing some light exercise, enjoying a healthy breakfast, and doing something calming like meditation or journalism. These activities work together to give you a great start to your day.

To boost your energy in the morning, try these easy tips. First, wake up at the same time every day so your body gets used to a regular sleep schedule. When you get up, drink a glass of water to help wake up your body.

Next, spend a few minutes stretching or doing some yoga to wake up your muscles and improve your flexibility. A healthy breakfast with protein and good fats can keep you feeling full of energy, so think about eating foods like eggs, avocados, or oatmeal. Finally, set aside some time to think about your day or plan out what you need to do. This can help you tackle any challenges with a clear mind and fresh motivation.

Creating a Nighttime Routine for Quality Sleep

A calming nighttime routine is really important for getting good sleep, which is key to your overall health. Having a steady routine tells your body it's time to wind down, helping you switch from the busyness of the day to a more relaxed state.

Some simple things to include in your calming evening routine are dimming the lights, doing relaxing activities like reading or taking a warm bath, and trying some mindfulness techniques to help quiet your mind.

To wind down well, think about setting a specific time for your nighttime routine that starts about an hour before you want to sleep. This means turning off electronic devices that give off blue light, which can mess with your sleep. Instead, choose calming activities like listening to soft music, writing in a gratitude journal, or doing some gentle stretches.

Making your sleep space comfortable—cool, dark, and quiet—will also help you fall asleep and stay asleep through the night. By making a soothing nighttime routine a priority, you'll boost your chances of getting restorative sleep, which can give you more energy and focus during the day.

Here's a table summarizing nutritional elements that can help improve sleep, based on the information provided:

Tracking Progress and Staying Consistent

Watching how you're doing with your health is a great way to stay inspired and on track as you work toward your wellness goals. Keeping track of your habits and results helps you see what works for you, find areas that could use some improvement, and celebrate your successes along the way.

You can use easy tools like notebooks, apps, or fitness trackers to monitor things like exercise, what you eat, and how well you sleep.

It's also key to stay motivated when things get tough. Everyone has challenges, but viewing them as part of your journey can help you keep going. Try to set small, achievable goals so you can see progress without feeling overwhelmed. Checking in on your goals regularly and celebrating your wins—big or small—can lift your spirits and help you form good habits. By adding tracking to your routine, you create a helpful system that keeps you consistent and healthy, especially after 40.

Ready to take charge of your health journey? Download our free Health Progress Tracking Checklist today! This useful tool will help you track your habits, stay motivated, and celebrate your wins every step of the way. Just click the link below to get started and make your wellness goals a reality!

Health and Wellness Checklist

1. Goal Setting
   Short-term Goals (1 month):

   - Weight: Target weight (e.g., lose 4 pounds)
   - Exercise: Number of workouts per week (e.g., 4 times)
   - Daily Steps: Target steps (e.g., 10,000 steps)
   - Water: Daily intake (e.g., 64 ounces)

   Long-term Goals (6 months):

   - Weight: Target weight (e.g., lose 20 pounds)
   - Fitness: Achieve a fitness goal (e.g., run a 5K)
   - Nutrition: Reduce sugar intake (e.g., below 25 grams/day)

2. Daily Exercise Tracking

- Workout Type (e.g., cardio, strength)
- Duration (e.g., 30 minutes)
- Intensity (e.g., light, moderate, vigorous)
- Daily Steps: Count of steps
- Personal Records (e.g., lifted X pounds)

3. Nutrition Monitoring

- Food Journal: Log meals and snacks
- Daily Calories: Total calories consumed
- Protein: Target (e.g., 100 grams/day)
- Carbs: Target (e.g., 150 grams/day)
- Fats: Target (e.g., 50 grams/day)
- Sugar: Daily intake
- Water: Ounces consumed

4. Sleep Patterns

- Bedtime: The time you go to bed
- Wake Time: The time you wake up
- Total Sleep: Hours slept (aim for 7-9)
- Sleep Quality: Rate on a scale of 1-10
- Nighttime Awakenings: Any disturbances

5. Mental Wellbeing

- Daily Mood: Rate mood (1-10)
- Daily Stress: Rate stress (1-10) and note stressors
- Mindfulness Practice:
- Type (e.g., meditation)
- Duration: Time spent

6. Weekly Reviews

- Weight Check: Weigh yourself
- Total Workouts: Number of workouts
- Total Steps: Count for the week
- Nutritional Review: Reflect on eating habits
- Adjust Goals: Update based on progress

7. Monthly Check-ins

- Progress Photos: Take pictures
- Measurements: Record body measurements
- Fitness Assessment: Re-evaluate goals
- Celebrate Achievements: Acknowledge milestones

8. Support and Accountability

- Accountability Partner: Find someone to check in with
- Join a Group: Look for support groups

Additional Tips:

- Be Consistent: Stick to your routine
- Focus on Progress: Celebrate small wins
- Use Tools: Try apps or journals that work for you

Feel free to print or keep this checklist handy to help you stay organized and motivated on your health journey!

Section 2: Overcoming Common Challenges

Going through midlife and focusing on health and wellness often comes with its own set of challenges that can slow you down. It's important to see these common obstacles and find ways to deal with them so you can keep making positive changes and enjoy a healthy lifestyle. In this section, we'll look at tips for breaking old habits, managing pressures from friends and family, and staying motivated while preventing burnout.

Breaking Through Old Habits

When things start to change, it's common for old habits to come back, which can get in the way of making progress. This can happen for a few reasons, like feeling comfortable with what you already know, emotional triggers, or stress that pulls you back into old ways. Understanding why these habits return is the first step to moving past them.

To break free from habits that don't help you, it's important to spot what triggers them and come up with ways to deal with those triggers. Start by being aware of yourself; try keeping a journal to note when and why your old habits pop up. This will give you a better idea of how to tackle those triggers with healthier choices.

Building new, good habits takes time and practice, so think about using the habit-stacking method. This means you link a new habit to something you already do. For instance, if you want to get into the habit of exercising, do it right after your morning routine. By focusing on small changes and treating yourself for little wins, you can gradually shift your thinking and replace old habits with better ones.

Handling Social and Family Pressures

Your journey to better health and well-being can sometimes be affected by what others say or expect, whether it's family, friends, or even coworkers. Comments, comparisons, or requests for changes in how you live can make it hard to focus on your own health goals and might leave you feeling guilty or unhappy. That's why clear communication is so important.

Let the people close to you know what your health goals are and why they matter to you. When you share your reasons, it helps them understand and support your choices. You might also think about forming a support group with friends or family who have similar health goals. This way, you can encourage each other and stay motivated.

Joining group activities and being around positive, supportive people can help reduce any negative pressure you feel. Remember, it's completely okay to speak up about your needs and prioritize your health; doing this not only benefits you but also inspires others to take care of themselves too!

Example:

You've decided to live a healthier life by focusing on better eating and regular exercise. At family gatherings, you notice that some relatives often offer you unhealthy snacks or question why you're not having dessert. Instead of feeling guilty or pressured, you decide to talk to your family about your health goals.

At the next family dinner, you say, "I'm working on my health because I want to feel more energetic and stay healthy as I get older. I'm trying to eat more nutritious foods and keep up with my workouts." By explaining your reasons, your family starts to understand your choices better.

Because of this, they begin to offer healthier options at meals and cheer you on with your exercise goals. Plus, you invite your sister to go for walks with you each week, helping both of you stay on track.

This open talk not only eases the pressure you felt before but also strengthens your family bonds as they join you on your health journey. By making your health a priority, you set a good example that encourages others to think about their well-being too.

Staying Motivated and Avoiding Burnout

As you work toward your health goals, it's crucial to recognize signs of goal fatigue or burnout. This can manifest as a lack of enthusiasm, increased irritability, or a sense of overwhelm. Staying motivated requires proactive strategies to keep your energy levels high and your focus sharp.

Implement techniques such as setting realistic and achievable goals, and breaking them down into smaller milestones that allow for a sense of accomplishment along the way. Engaging in regular self-reflection can also help you reassess your goals and align them with your evolving needs and values.

When motivation begins to wane, rekindle your passion by revisiting your original "why"—the reasons you started this journey in the first place. Connecting back to your motivation can reignite your commitment and drive.

Incorporating variety into your routine can also combat monotony and burnout. Experiment with new activities, recipes, or workout classes to keep things fresh and exciting. Finally, prioritize self-care to ensure you're nurturing both your physical and mental health. By taking proactive steps to maintain motivation and avoid burnout, you can overcome challenges and sustain your journey toward a vibrant and healthy midlife.

If you don't break your larger goals into smaller milestones or set hard but achievable goals, you may encounter several negative outcomes that can hinder your progress:

1. **Feeling frustrated and overwhelmed**: Without smaller goals, working toward your big health goals can seem too hard. When you don't see progress, it's easy to feel stuck and lose track of what you want to achieve.
2. **Losing motivation**: When you reach small goals, it gives you a sense of success and lifts your spirits. If you skip these little wins, you might feel like you're not moving forward, which can take away your excitement and commitment to getting healthy.
3. **Burnout risk**: Setting goals that are too big without breaking them down into smaller steps can lead to burnout. Trying to be perfect all the time without celebrating your progress can be tiring and may make you want to give up on your health habits altogether.
4. **Not taking time to reflect**: If you don't regularly check in on your goals, you might find they don't match what you really need or care about anymore. This disconnect can make it hard to stay motivated since you might be chasing after goals that no longer matter to you.
5. **Losing accountability**: Smaller goals create good chances for you to check in on yourself and adjust your plans if needed. If you skip these steps, you might miss moments to hold yourself accountable and track your progress, which makes it harder to stick with your health journey.

Section 3: Building a Supportive Environment

Making a supportive environment is important for promoting health and wellness, especially during midlife when so much is changing. The places we live, the people we spend time with, and the communities we are part of can have a big impact on our motivation, feelings, and overall health. In this section, we'll look at some simple ways to create a healthy living space, find someone to help keep you on track with your health goals and connect with a community to support your wellness journey.

Creating a Healthy Living Space

Your home is the base for your daily life and can either help or make it harder to reach your health goals. A neat and calm living space can create a sense of peace and focus, which is important for making positive changes.

Start by clearing out clutter, as a tidy space can help clear your mind. Use storage solutions to keep items in the right places, which can reduce distractions.

Add things that boost your well-being, like plants that improve air quality and bring a bit of nature inside. Set up cozy spots for relaxation, like a reading corner or a quiet place for meditation, where you can unwind and recharge.

Think about how lighting affects your mood; natural light can brighten your spirits, so try to let in as much as possible by opening curtains during the day or using warm light bulbs in the evening. By making these simple changes to your home, you can create an environment that supports wellness, encourages mindfulness, and helps you reach your health goals.

Finding a Health Accountability Partner

Having a health accountability partner can provide the encouragement and motivation needed to stay committed to your wellness goals. This partnership involves regularly checking in with each other, sharing progress, and holding each other accountable for maintaining healthy habits.

To choose a supportive partner, look for someone who shares similar goals or values but may be at a different point in their journey. This dynamic can create a balanced partnership where both individuals can learn from each other.

Communication is vital in this relationship. Set clear expectations regarding how often you'll check in and what form those interactions will take, whether through phone calls, texts, or in-person meetings. Be open about your challenges and victories, fostering an environment of honesty and support.

To enhance the effectiveness of your partnership, consider setting joint goals, participating in activities together, or attending wellness events. By supporting each other's goals and celebrating achievements, you'll build a strong foundation of encouragement that can propel both of you toward success.

Connecting with a Community

Having social support is important during midlife and can greatly improve your health and happiness. Being part of a community gives you chances to share experiences, make friends, and find motivation, which can help you stay focused on your wellness journey.

Look for local or online wellness groups that match your interests, whether that's fitness, nutrition, or general health. Many community centers, gyms, and health organizations offer classes or support groups designed for specific needs and groups of people.

Try joining activities that promote physical health and help you connect with others, like group fitness classes, walking clubs, or workshops. If you can't find local options, check out online platforms where you can meet people with similar interests, join discussions, and share helpful resources.

Also, think about volunteering for causes you care about, as this can give you a sense of purpose and help you meet new people. By looking for connections in your community, you can boost your emotional well-being, share helpful tips, and build lasting friendships that make your midlife journey even better.

Chapter 4: Embracing Your Best Self Beyond 40

Section 1: Redefining Success and Happiness

Stepping into midlife gives you a special chance to rethink what success and happiness mean for you. With a better understanding of yourself and what's important, this time can be filled with growth, fulfillment, and self-discovery. Becoming your best self after 40 means looking at your values, setting new and meaningful goals, and finding joy in everyday moments. Here are some ways you can create a life that matches your changing sense of purpose and happiness.

Reflecting on Personal Values

As we get older, our values can change based on our experiences, relationships, and how we see the world. Midlife is a great time to think about these changes and how they influence the life you want to live.

Take a moment to pause and think about what's important to you now. What makes you feel fulfilled? What gives you a sense of peace or pride? Your answers might be different from what mattered to you when you were younger, and that's completely normal.

Try some activities to help you understand your current values better. You could write in a journal about meaningful experiences from your past or think about the qualities you admire in other people. You might also want to create a list of your values and narrow it down to your top five.

Looking at these values can help you line up your goals, daily choices, and actions with what truly matters to you, giving you a greater sense of purpose and direction.

Setting New, Meaningful Goals

Redefining success in midlife can be incredibly freeing, allowing you to set goals that resonate with your inner values rather than external expectations. Rather than pursuing achievements that may not bring personal fulfillment, focus on setting goals that feel genuinely meaningful.

Think about what makes you feel alive and purposeful, whether that's personal development, nurturing relationships, or pursuing passions.

Start by creating a vision of the person you want to become, considering the areas where you'd like to grow or learn. Then, set goals that support this vision, ensuring they're specific, realistic, and aligned with your values.

For example, if family and relationships are important to you, setting a goal to spend quality time with loved ones each week can create a positive shift. Write down your goals and break them into manageable steps, making it easier to track progress and stay motivated. As you make strides toward these meaningful goals, you'll find yourself embracing success that feels more authentic and fulfilling.

Personal Development Checklist

1. Define Your Core Values

- Identify and write down your top three personal values (e.g., family, health, creativity).

____

____

____

2. Set a Personal Development Goal

- Choose one skill to develop this year (e.g., learn a new language, take a cooking class).
- Outline three specific steps to achieve this goal:
- Step 1: ______________________

- Step 2: ___________________________
- Step 3: ___________________________

3. Enhance Relationships

- Schedule a weekly family night (e.g., every Friday) to strengthen connections.
- Plan activities in advance to make it special: ________________________

4. Pursue a Passion Project

- Identify one passion (e.g., painting, gardening).
- Commit to dedicating at least one hour each week to this passion: ___________________________

5. Reflect and Adjust Goals

- Set a reminder to review your goals every three months.
- Assess your progress and make adjustments as needed:
- Next review date: ___________________________
- Notes for adjustments: ___________________________

Feel free to print this checklist or keep it somewhere you can easily see it to help you stay focused on your goals!

Finding Joy in Everyday Moments

In the pursuit of goals, it's easy to overlook the small, joyful moments that make life beautiful. Practicing mindfulness can help you slow down and appreciate life's simple pleasures, from a warm cup of tea to a heartfelt conversation. By bringing attention to these moments, you cultivate a deeper sense of gratitude and joy.

Incorporate practices that invite more joy into your daily life. Take a few minutes each day to savor something you love, like watching the sunrise, enjoying a favorite meal, or reading a book.

Make a habit of acknowledging moments of happiness, however brief, and allowing yourself to be fully present in them. Another helpful practice is to end each day by reflecting on three positive experiences, reinforcing your appreciation for life's everyday gifts.

Embracing these small moments nurtures a contentment that enriches both your inner and outer life, helping you live more joyfully and meaningfully in midlife and beyond.

In the pursuit of goals, it's easy to overlook the small, joyful moments that make life beautiful. Practicing mindfulness can help you slow down and appreciate life's simple pleasures, from a warm cup of tea to a heartfelt conversation. By bringing attention to these moments, you cultivate a deeper sense of gratitude and joy.

Incorporate practices that invite more joy into your daily life. For me, I spend time each day reading novels, which allows me to escape into different worlds and savor the stories. If I still feel off after that, I'll go out for a walk, often in the garden, just to let myself explore the outdoors. Seeing people, feeling the sun on my skin, and embracing the fresh air adds a rejuvenating element to my day.

Make a habit of acknowledging moments of happiness, however brief, and allowing yourself to be fully present in them. Another helpful practice is to end each day by reflecting on three positive experiences, reinforcing your appreciation for life's everyday gifts. Embracing these small moments nurtures a contentment that enriches both your inner and outer life, helping you live more joyfully and meaningfully in midlife and beyond.

Section 2: Fostering a Growth Mindset

Developing a growth mindset in midlife can be a transformative journey, opening up opportunities for continuous growth, resilience, and fulfillment. Embracing lifelong learning, adaptability, and resilience enables you to navigate life's changes with confidence and turn challenges into moments of growth. Here's how to foster a mindset that will empower you to thrive beyond 40.

The Power of Lifelong Learning

Lifelong learning adds energy and curiosity to our lives, and it's especially helpful as we reach midlife. Trying out new things keeps our minds active, sparks creativity, and helps us adjust to changes.

For me, I enjoy exploring healthy cooking by learning new dishes that taste good and nourish my body. I love experimenting with different ingredients and finding recipes that fit my health goals. I'm also interested in learning how to make money online.

The online world is always changing, and I have fun taking courses and tutorials that teach me the skills I need to create opportunities for myself. Whether it's through blogging, freelancing, or trying out e-commerce, I find excitement in all the possibilities.

You can also find joy in learning, whether it's picking up a new hobby, diving into a topic you've always wanted to explore, or improving your job skills. Think about subjects that interest you, like learning a new language, getting into photography, or studying health and nutrition.

To make learning a part of your daily life, start by setting aside just 15 minutes each day to read, watch tutorials, or practice a new skill. Online courses and local workshops can help you learn in a structured way, while simple habits like reading daily or listening to educational podcasts make learning easy and rewarding.

Over time, developing a love for learning can be energizing, helping you feel more engaged and capable in every part of your life.

Embracing Change and Adaptability

Midlife often brings a lot of changes, whether it's in your career, family life, or personal priorities. Being open and flexible with these changes can help you move forward more easily.

Being resilient doesn't mean you ignore the tough parts of change. It means facing them with a flexible and open mindset. Looking at each transition as a chance to grow can help lower stress and make the journey feel more rewarding.

To become more adaptable, start by making small changes to your routine or trying new challenges. This can help you feel more comfortable with change. Simple practices like meditation or journaling can keep you grounded during uncertain times, and setting flexible goals can give you direction without feeling too strict.

Look at each change as an opportunity to learn something new, and keep in mind that being adaptable is a skill you can improve over time. When you face change with an open mind, you'll be more ready for the shifts that life brings your way.

Turning Setbacks into Opportunities

Setbacks are a regular part of life, and midlife brings challenges and surprises. A growth mindset means seeing these setbacks not as failures, but as chances to learn and get better. When you look at challenges this way, you can become more resilient, understand yourself better, and feel more confident when facing future problems.

To see setbacks as opportunities, take a moment to think about what each challenge teaches you. Writing in a journal about what went well, what you could do better, and how you handled the situation can give you valuable insights.

Look at the setback as a stepping stone and think about the skills or strengths you gained from it. Positively handling tough times can make you more resilient, helping you become stronger and ready for life's challenges. Seeing each challenge as a chance to grow can lead to a more satisfying and resilient life after 40.

Section 3: Celebrating Your Journey and Looking Forward

Reaching midlife brings a wealth of experiences, accomplishments, and wisdom worth celebrating. Embracing your journey is about recognizing your progress, setting a hopeful vision for the future, and finding meaningful ways to share what you've learned. This chapter encourages you to look back with pride, look forward with intention, and enrich both your life and others through giving back.

Acknowledging Your Progress

Celebrating progress, no matter how big or small, is essential to maintaining motivation and self-confidence. Reflecting on your achievements—whether they are career milestones, personal growth, or even moments of resilience during challenging times—provides a sense of accomplishment and reinforces your strength.

Recognizing these wins can be as simple as journaling about your successes each month or sharing milestones with close friends or family. Try dedicating time each week to review what you've achieved, from small daily wins to significant milestones, and give yourself credit for the journey so far.

Reflection exercises, like writing down three things you're proud of each day, help you stay connected to your progress and encourage continued growth.

Celebrating these accomplishments not only boosts your confidence but also helps maintain a positive outlook. Each step forward, no matter how minor, represents resilience and perseverance, creating a foundation for future growth.

Planning for a Vibrant Future

I wish I could still look as young as I am now after 10 years, and wish I will have better strength after 10 years, that's why I'm maintaining a healthy diet & exercising at home daily.

Setting intentions for a vibrant future provides motivation and direction. In midlife, you have the unique opportunity to design a future aligned with your true values and goals. Envision what you want the next decade to look like, considering not only physical health but also emotional and mental well-being.

For me, this means committing to a well-rounded fitness routine that includes strength training, flexibility exercises, and cardio workouts. I also prioritize meal planning each week, ensuring I incorporate a variety of nutrient-rich foods that support my overall health.

Perhaps you envision a decade filled with new adventures, meaningful relationships, or creative pursuits that bring you joy and fulfillment. Defining this vision helps keep you inspired and focused on your aspirations.

Consider creating a "vision board" or journaling about your goals for the years ahead, whether they involve travel, learning new skills, or building deeper connections with loved ones. Setting specific milestones, like achieving a certain level of fitness or trying a new healthy recipe each week, allows me to track my progress.

Set intentions to prioritize wellness, growth, and joy, and

revisit these intentions regularly to stay motivated. This future-oriented mindset encourages hope and excitement, turning each day into a step toward a meaningful and fulfilling life.

Sharing Wisdom and Giving Back

Sharing your experiences and knowledge not only helps others but also gives you a sense of purpose. Think about what you've learned and how you can share it, whether it's through mentoring, volunteering, or supporting those on similar paths.

Mentoring younger coworkers or sharing life lessons with friends and family can be very rewarding. It helps build stronger connections and offers guidance to those facing challenges you've already dealt with.

Giving back can take many forms, from getting involved in your community to simply offering advice to a friend. This not only helps those you support but also improves your well-being, making you feel more connected and fulfilled.

Acts of giving encourage gratitude, keep you in touch with your values and add purpose to your day. By sharing your journey, you turn your experiences into a source of strength and inspiration, leaving a legacy that goes beyond just your achievements.

Conclusion

As we hit the big 4-0, many women start to face a bunch of health challenges, both mental and physical. This time in life can bring changes that feel a bit overwhelming, but it also offers a wonderful chance for growth and change. By focusing on our health and well-being, we can handle this journey with confidence and strength.

In this book, we've looked at different ways to boost your health and energy during midlife. We talked about redefining what success means to you, setting meaningful goals, and taking care of both your body and mind. Each chapter was packed with tips and insights to help you feel empowered on this path. We highlighted the importance of self-care, the benefits of learning throughout life, and the value of building supportive relationships. By adding these ideas to your daily routine, you can create a lively and fulfilling life that truly reflects who you are.

I want to take a moment to thank you for reading this book and for taking the time to focus on your well-being. Your dedication to improving your health and embracing this new chapter is inspiring, and I hope the ideas shared here motivate you to take control of your journey.

If you found this book helpful, I'd appreciate it if you could *leave a review on Amazon*. Your feedback not only helps me get better but also helps others find useful resources on their wellness journey. Thanks again for your support, and I wish you joy, strength, and a renewed sense of vitality on your path!

Resources

Weiss, R. V., Hohl, A., Athayde, A., Pardini, D., Gomes, L., De Oliveira, M., Meirelles, R., Clapauch, R., & Spritzer, P. M. (2019). Testosterone therapy for women with low sexual desire: a position statement from the Brazilian Society of Endocrinology and Metabolism. *Archives of Endocrinology and Metabolism, 63*(3), 190–198. https://doi.org/10.20945/2359-3997000000152

Glick, I. D., & Bennett, S. E. (1981). Psychiatric complications of progesterone and oral contraceptives*. *Journal of Clinical Psychopharmacology, 1*(6), 350–367. https://doi.org/10.1097/0 0004714-198111000-00003

Davis, S. R., Castelo-Branco, C., Chedraui, P., Lumsden, M. A., Nappi, R. E., Shah, D., & Villaseca, P. (2012). Understanding weight gain at menopause. *Climacteric, 15*(5), 419–429. https://doi.org/10.3109/13697137.2012.707385

Haufe, A., & Leeners, B. (2023). Sleep disturbances across a woman's lifespan: What is the role of reproductive hormones?

Journal of the Endocrine Society, 7(5). https://doi.org/10.1210/je
ndso/bvad036

Sunyecz, J. (2008). The use of calcium and vitamin D in the
management of osteoporosis. *Therapeutics and Clinical Risk
Management, Volume 4,* 827–836. https://doi.org/10.2147/tcr
m.s3552

Machuca, J. N., & Rosales-Alvarez, C. P. (2024). Cardiovascular
disease in women and the role of hormone replacement therapy.
Cureus. https://doi.org/10.7759/cureus.69752

Draelos, Z. D. (2011c). A clinical evaluation of the comparable
efficacy of hyaluronic acid-based foam and ceramide-
containing emulsion cream in the treatment of mild-to-
moderate atopic dermatitis. *Journal of Cosmetic Dermatology,
10*(3), 185–188. https://doi.org/10.1111/j.1473-2165.2011.00
568.x

Leeuwendaal, N. K., Stanton, C., O'Toole, P. W., & Beresford,
T. P. (2022). Fermented foods, health and the gut microbiome.
Nutrients, 14(7), 1527. https://doi.org/10.3390/nu14071527

Zone 2 training for AFIB patients. (n.d.). Dr. Andrea Tordini.
https://www.flheartbeat.com/zone-2-training-an-exercise-fo
r-most-afib-patients/#:~:text=Zone%20two%20training%2C%

20as%20it,fibrillation%20and%20other%20cardiovascular%20
concerns

Pattnaik, H., Mir, M., Boike, S., Kashyap, R., Khan, S. A., & Surani, S. (2022). Nutritional elements in sleep. *Cureus*. https://doi.org/10.7759/cureus.32803